Sweet, Sweet Sleep.

# Acknowledgements

I would like to thank my wife, Princess M, and my two wingers for giving me the inspiration and time to complete this book. I would also like to thank Coach Phyllis for her insight and time she gave to me during the writing. I can't forget to thank all my clients who I have learned a great deal from and continue to do. Thank you . . . sleep well.

I also recommend you check out my website at http://liferightsideup.com/ for more information.

# Table of Contents

# Preface

When I started my personal training business in 1996, I soon realized after spending just a short time with new clients that lack of sleep was more the norm than the exception. For most of my clients the dysfunctional sleep patterns had become so normal that the client rarely initiated the topic of sleep.

Coincidently these were the same clients who also struggled to meet their health goals. Whether it was weight loss, becoming stronger, or having more energy. This lead me to implementing a question about their sleep habits early in our first meeting.

This book covers the story of four clients who struggle with sleep. Within these stories are the most common problems I've seen over the last twenty years and the strategies used to combat them.

This book is different in that it will look at the rarely mentioned aspect of stress hormones and their intimate relation to poor sleep. The book will help you understand the why and get to the root of the problem.

Once a person normalizes their sleep habits they quickly recognize that their previous energy was indeed deficient.

It appears that sleep problems have become socially acceptable with some even wearing it as a badge of honor with that badge saying, "I can function on little sleep."

Did you know that 40 percent of people suffer from sleep problems? This is a scary fact. In 2010, it cost the United States' economy more than 63 billion dollars in health problems, work days missed, and low productivity.

This book will address at least two groups in the general population:

- Those who have difficulty falling asleep

- Those who wake in the middle of the night and struggle getting back to sleep

Various strategies are used by those suffering sleep problems. When people are deprived of this primal need, desperate times can call for desperate measures. Sleeping pills, alcohol, medication, and loud TV are examples of what some will try. This book looks at the causes of poor sleep because the physiological influence is more prominent than most believe. I believe to fix any problem the cause must first be known. More importantly, this book will offer you nutritional and lifestyle strategies which will result in a sound night's sleep.

*Sleep is the golden chain that ties health and our bodies together.*

— Thomas Dekker

Since starting my personal training business I have changed my view on many things regarding exercise, nutrition, and how I train and coach my clients. The methodology I use today is not something found in a grocery store aisle or on infomercials. It has come from much trial and error and from extensive study in exercise and nutritional prescription. I encourage readers to question me, but to also question their own present belief systems and ask themselves if it is serving them.

Reading, researching, and experimenting with sleep difficulty over the years, I have rarely found anything that dealt with the nocturnal hormones. Being able to control those hormones will result in controlling a good night's sleep.

Please see this book as a sleep reference book . . . your go-to book for a good night's sleep.

This book will take you through conversations with clients who suffer insomnia. You will see how the lifestyle changes I suggest and that clients implement positively impact not only their sleep, but their overall quality of life.

The anonymity of these clients has been changed, but the situations are real and very common.

*The true method of knowledge is experiment.*

— William Blake

# Judy

"I need your help!"

That was the message left on my phone. Judy had gotten my name from another client and wanted to set up an appointment. I returned Judy's call and she briefly described how she had just turned 60 and wanted to "get in shape." She said she wanted to lose some inches and had no background in weight training. Two things typically stand out in the first call. First, the potential client has usually had a recent birthday ending in zero; and second, they are typically vague about their goals until more questions are directed their way.

I emailed Judy my assessment sheets to fill out and set up an appointment. The email I sent dealt with questions about digestion, hormones, limbic and nervous systems to name a few. To arrive at the root cause of certain problems, however, a full assessment is required. "If you are not assessing, you are guessing," a teacher once said.

The questionnaire also weeds out people who may or may not be serious about the program. I received notice that she completed the questionnaire on the same day, so I started forming a mental picture of how this person's lifestyle appeared. Typically, for women over the age of about thirty-five, hormonal issues are at the root of the problem.

*Women suffer from 75 percent of all autoimmune diseases which would strongly suggest that hormones are a major influence in a variety of issues.*

The questionnaire showed Judy scored high in the hormonal zone which wasn't ideal. This was not uncommon nor was the fact her sleep quality, digestion, muscle, and joint pain scores were moderate to high as well.

A week later I met Judy at her house and it was time to ask more questions. Judy, semi-retired from a business she had started thirty years ago, was now looking to invest in herself. After getting the tour of her workout room we headed to the kitchen.

"Judy, what are your goals?" I asked as we settled at the table.

"I want to look like I did when I was twenty!" She said and laughed. "But seriously, I just want to have more energy and keep doing the things I love to do like gardening and golfing without injury. I mentioned losing some body fat on the phone but that would truly be a bonus."

I believe as a coach the questions should outweigh the answers so I asked, "What will it take for you to get to that place?"

"You need to kick my ass in shape!" she laughed.

"That's one way," I said. "Stress can indeed force things to grow but if your flowers were dehydrated and had no sunshine would throwing some bugs on them help or add to the problem?"

"Are you saying I'm stressed?" Judy asked. "Do you think I'm stressed?"

"Like your flowers there are all different forms of stress," I answered. "Stress can be physical, emotional, mental, and environmental to name just a few. These can have an accumulative effect on the body, and over time, sickness or disease may be the end result."

I had a copy of her questionnaire with me which I placed on the table.

"How is your sleep?" I asked.

"Horrible, but who sleeps well? Even my doctor said that was normal and offered me sleeping pills or antidepressants but I just laughed at him. So he recommended some exercise which is one of the reasons I called you. You have to fix me," she pleaded.

"How long has your sleep been bothering you?" I asked.

"Oh, about ten years I would imagine," Judy admitted.

"Is it a problem falling to sleep or is it waking during the night?"

"Most of the time I fall asleep quickly but then wake and I'm wide awake tossing and turning and throwing the sheets off. I'm afraid to look at the clock. I probably lay there for an hour or more before I get back to sleep. Sometimes I don't get back to sleep," Judy sighed.

Even though this was a fact finding session, I try to give my clients some useful information to leave with and apply before our next session.

"Judy, do you know what your resting pulse is during the day?" I asked.

"On my last visit to the doctor he told me it was . . . seventy . . . but lately my memory is not the best."

"Ok, so we have a reference point during the night if you wake. If you wake and feel you can't or won't get back to sleep anytime soon then I want you to take your pulse again either physically yourself or use something like an oximeter or phone app."

"Are you writing this down? Don't forget my bad memory," Judy said.

"Duly noted. I will give you notes for any homework."

"Why do want me to check my heart rate?"

"The test is to check if adrenaline and possibly cortisol are driving the problems of your restless sleep. A person's pulse typically drops about 8 to 10 percent during sleep. If your heart rate is elevated, we know adrenaline and likely cortisol are involved. We can then try to manage those hormones with food," I explained.

"Is it chocolate? Please let it be chocolate."

"I get a feeling you like chocolate Judy."

"I crave chocolate but I know that's bad," Judy said.

"I don't like to say any food is good or bad. All foods have a place in the right context. I don't like to demonize any particular food but we can go over that next time."

I told Judy that before we meet next time I wanted her to monitor her resting heart rate at least twice a day. I told her if she awoke during the night to record it and first thing in the morning too.

"Sometimes during the night, the increase can be so noticeable that you feel like your heart is pounding through your chest," I told her.

Judy nodded in agreement.

I handed her some sheets and said, "I also want you to record at least five days of eating and include the weekend because some people can go off the rails a little on the weekend."

"Guilty as charged," she said, laughing.

Reaching for my jacket I continued, "The next time we meet, we will talk about nutrition and I'll take you through some physical assessments. How does that sound?"

Judy replied, "Looking forward to it . . . I think."

I try not to overload a client with homework or information in the first meeting because most people already have too much on their proverbial plate.

A week later I arrived at Judy's for the physical assessment part of the program.

I had just laid my bag down when Judy blurted, "My heart rates were up!"

"You mean when you would wake during the night?" I asked.

"Yeah, is that what's supposed to happen?" she asked with concern in her voice.

"It's not really what is supposed to happen, but it's what I had expected and why I had you do that homework," I said. "You already had the baseline of seventy bpm from your doctor so having an elevated heart rate explains why you are waking.

I explained to Judy that one of the driving factors of the increased heart rate is the darkness of night. Darkness can be extremely stressful to the body evidenced in the fact that death rates increase during months with shorter daylight hours and may also explain why most deaths occur during night.

"I can't leave the lights on," Judy said. "That would drive me crazy!"

"No, no, that's not ideal either. Our sleep is supposed to counteract this stressor if we do indeed sleep," I said. "Judy, what do you eat or drink before going to bed?"

"I try not to eat anything. I saw some health expert on TV talking about calories turning to fat when eaten late and eating late can disrupt your sleep or so I thought."

"Having something before bed may affect sleep, but it is more dependent on exactly what it is you eat that will have a positive or negative effect."

Grinning I asked, "Judy, how does having something sweet and salty appeal to you just before bed?"

"Oh dear, that would be lovely, but I don't want to gain fat, if I haven't mentioned that already," she said as she pinched her side and winked.

"If we look at the fact that you are not sleeping solidly, then that alone can cause body fat to accumulate," I told her. "When the stress hormone cortisol consistently stays elevated then body fat may be deposited."

"I don't want that!"

"What can occur during the night is that the stress hormones of cortisol and adrenaline elevate and cause you to wake. The darkness of night contributes to this, but also what you have or haven't eaten during the day can play a large factor. The hormone of estrogen can play an additional huge role in sleep disruption," I explained.

"No worries about estrogen because I have already gone through menopause so my estrogen should be low," Judy said.

I replied, "What is more important is the estrogen to progesterone ratio."

I continued to teach Judy as she listened attentively. I told her that even if blood tests show estrogen to be normal for that lab, the progesterone still needs to be higher. Blood tests don't show the estrogen that has accumulated in a tissue like the breast or uterus. Estrogen can have an impact on blood sugar handling and this causes that hormone cortisol mentioned earlier to rise.

Keeping cortisol levels under control can help with sleep, but also prevent many degenerative diseases.

After a long pause, Judy replied, "All right, let me get this straight. You are saying the avoidance of food before bed, the darkness, and the estrogen all affect the adrenaline and corti...."

"Cortisol."

"Right, cortisol," Judy answered. "Would those hormones affect my joints in the morning too?"

"Possibly. Once you start sleeping correctly your rate of physical breakdown slows and that should affect a lot of other factors," I clarified.

"Geez, I never really thought about it that way. It has been going on so long I just accepted it as normal. It has been quite the norm for me and most of my friends."

I nodded, saying, "Ok, I have some homework for you before our session next week. I want you to try a salt and sugar 'Night Nog'."

Judy smiled, "I get to drink wine and eat chips?"

"Not exactly, but hormones can cause some people to reach for those food choices."

One of the "Night Nogs," or "brews," consists of a teaspoon of honey, a teaspoon of unflavored coconut oil, and a pinch of white refined sea salt dissolved in three to four ounces of hot water and then topped off with four to five more ounces of white milk. As I shared the recipe, Judy looked at me with surprise and doubt.

This is a common reaction when I tell clients to add (sea) salt to their diet, and something sweet.

"Oil in milk?" Judy scrunched her lips indicating dislike.

I laughed, "I know! That choice doesn't appeal to everyone. You can try it without the oil if you like."

"Like all my suggestions, I recommend people trying it first and not let cultural and programmed beliefs creep into your decisions. If it doesn't work, then you call me crazy and you may be in search for a new trainer," I said smiling.

Judy responded, "Well what I'm doing now isn't working so something needs to change."

"That's the type of practical intellect I like to hear," I said.

After I finished the physical assessments I gave her some physical homework (which were exercise and stretches) and gathered her food logs to study.

A week later I arrived at her house and was greeted by an energetic Judy.

"Well I took your Night Nogs faithfully during the week," she said with an excited look.

"How did it go?"

"It went really well! I slept solid. I had one night when I had a couple glasses of wine and woke up feeling hot around 2 a.m. Would the wine have caused that reaction?" She asked.

"It's common to get that reaction from alcohol," I said.

"Well I rarely drink so I'm willing to trade a drink for the occasional disrupted sleep," Judy smirked. "You will be so proud of me. I even added unflavoured coconut oil and I was surprised it wasn't too bad. Do you have other suggestions for night time Nogs?" she asked.

"I do indeed. Those who have a hard time with milk can also substitute orange juice with a shake of sea salt in it. Orange juice can be very effective."

Depending on the person, the addition of salt is always optional.

"The orange juice should be pulp free and not from concentrate." I continued, "Some of these companies enzymatically change the pulp which is why it floats and can lead to digestive problems."

"Oh dear, I don't want that."

"Concentrated drinks will tend to blend the complete fruit and seeds into the drink which can cause intestinal distress."

"That sounds nasty."

"If you do find pulp free orange juice hard on digestion, you can try adding about a ¼ teaspoon of baking soda to it to diminish the acid or have some cheese alongside. Some clients actually find a different brand of orange juice or other tropical juice easier on their digestion."

"Is this some sort of black magic drink you have created to knock people out?" Judy asked, smiling.

I laughed. "Actually, it has a solid basis in how the body works."

I had already shared with Judy how the body secretes the stress hormones adrenaline and cortisol commonly at night due to the darkness and low glycogen levels. Those hormones rise when the body is running low on stored energy (glycogen). The body's emergency response system activates adrenaline and cortisol into action to break down parts of the body like the tissues, organs, and bones needed for fuel. When the adrenaline rises so does the heart rate and the result is being woke up.

"Is that why I need the juice, Sean?"

"Exactly," I said. "The orange juice contains glucose and fructose which is a form of sugar, and the milk has lactose with honey adding the glucose and fructose. The sugar will tend to keep cortisol and adrenaline levels down while the salt also lowers adrenaline."

Judy nodded. "But how about my blood pressure?"

"Always consult your doctor when making changes. With the addition of salt especially for those who intentionally restrict sodium there may be some fluid retention the first few days while the body adapts. I'm not saying to pour it on everything you eat but cravings are a good indicator of what the body needs. People who crave salty foods like potato chips or olives usually are missing their salt and are trying to compensate for it elsewhere."

"I love potato chips," Judy said.

"No doubt, the need for salt can vary. Circumstances like climate and physical activity levels will affect cravings too."

I explained that problems arise with cravings when we crave sugar but reach for cake and cookies. They can give immediate energy but are not the ideal foods for restoring long-term energy to the body. A person with low energy usually has sleep problems and vice versa. Eating the right foods and combination of foods will have a very positive effect on energy and sleep. The Night Nogs will help many people immediately, but keeping the liver, brain, and muscles supplied with enough glycogen (sugar) will produce long-term benefits and not just in the sleep category.

"Judy, I noticed you sometimes go five to six hours without eating. I only have a snapshot of one week, but is this a typical week for you?"

"Unfortunately, I'd have to say yes."

I continued, "Eating frequently or 'grazing' as some people call it can go a long way in maintaining blood sugar levels. If blood sugar drops then cortisol will elevate and that stress hormone is something you want relatively low most of the time. This is also where food cravings tend to spring up and we reach for foods that have low nutrient value."

"You are describing me."

"Planning is very important, but not to the point it becomes obsessive. I'm trying to lower the stressors in your life. I'm not trying to add to them. Cooking extra for supper and having leftovers for lunch is a great way to avoid unwanted meals at lunch. Having a mid-morning and mid-afternoon snack can also help. Many of my clients have a few ounces of milk or orange juice or a combination of both throughout the day."

"Milk and orange juice together?" Judy asked.

"Right."

"That's gross!"

"Have you tried it?"

"Heavens no."

"Judy, would it be fair to say this is an example of where the mind is winning over the body?"

Judy grimaced, "But milk and orange juice?"

"Judy, the clients who seem to have the most road blocks are usually also the ones who are slaves to their minds."

"What do you mean exactly?"

"Judy, did you use Windows 98 when it was first available"?

"I believe I did."

"When that system became outdated and didn't serve you anymore, did you upgrade to something that works better?"

"Gotcha. I see your point, Sean."

"I'm not singling out the orange juice and the milk combination because that's not a mandatory change. Nothing I say is mandatory. These are recommendations that should put you on the right path."

"Then it's up to me to walk down the path."

"Exactly."

"How does the rest of the food log look?" she asked.

"Well there is no one food protocol for everyone. Some people think weight loss and health are synonymous," I told her. "Your energy, mood, sleep quality, skin quality, digestion, hormones, libido and physical functioning would represent your health status better than a number on a scale."

I continued, "So, what I would recommend is that you try not to go more than four hours without food and when you do eat, try to have some combination of carbs, protein, and fat."

"Like what?"

"An example would be an omelet cooked in butter and some fruit for breakfast with the fruit being the carb, the egg being the protein, and the butter and yolk supplying the fat," I said.

"Sounds like something I'd enjoy eating."

"If you enjoy it you will be more likely to stick to it right?"

"Oh yes!"

"Healthy eating shouldn't be about deprivation and self-torture."

"Good point. How about lunch?" Judy asked.

"Lunch could be leftovers like some fish or meat with stir-fry vegetables cooked in coconut oil. Again, the veggies are the carb, the fish the protein, and the coconut oil is the fat."

Judy smirked. "You sure like your coconut oil."

"Our bodies deserve the best don't you think?"

Judy nodded.

"Supper could be your choice of meat or fish with some baked potatoes in butter. If your diet contains plenty of fruit and dairy, then things should go very well. If you eat 80 percent of the time what the body needs, then you should be able to handle a 20 percent 'assault'."

"I mentioned salt earlier and I do tell people to listen to their cravings in that regard," I told her. "Fruit or juice with some protein and fat alongside it can have a blood sugar stabilizing effect on the body. The fat and protein from cheese would be a good source or just having milk which also has a good combination of carbs, protein, and fat to maintain level blood sugar. High consumption of fruit is great because of the high potassium and fructose content both of which will have a powerful influence on regulating blood sugar. Some people choose the gluten-free version thinking it's healthier, but that version will still have added gums. Most people only eat about nine different foods so expanding the choices away from our safety and security can be difficult."

I gave Judy her home program and we set up another meeting in a few weeks to re-evaluate.

Three weeks later I showed up at Judy's house.

"How's everything going?" I asked with some anticipation.

"Great!" she said, excitedly. "I haven't slept this well in years! My energy is better the next day and my mood is much more stable. I also don't have the same level of cravings that I had before. I didn't think my cravings would change."

"That could definitely be related to better sleep. Rarely does someone wake up from sleep or a nap and have immediate cravings. The consumption of fruit, milk, or fruit juices throughout the day will play a big role too," I said.

"Well," Judy said. "I haven't been perfect, but much improved. I have found my muscles and joints aching less, too, so I guess my total stressors are starting to lower," she said with a big smile.

"That's great news Judy."

"The newfound energy has even given me incentive to walk thirty minutes a day!" Judy now seemingly stood taller.

"Wow, that is impressive!"

"I'm trying to put my new energy to good use," she said.

"Remember," I said. "This is a process, and everybody needs to keep listening to their body and fine tuning to what works well for them. Most people do very well with the addition of the

Night Nogs before bed and not going to bed on an empty stomach."

"Well, this is agreeing with my body," Judy said contently. "By the way, I told my good friend Mary about your Night Nogs and she said she tried them and had some success, but still has had some problems sleeping. She is planning on calling you to arrange an appointment," Judy said.

"Well I look forward to meeting her and look forward to your progress too Judy."

"Me too!" Judy said.

## Judy's Keys to Success

- **Obtaining a baseline of her resting heart rate during day and comparing it to her awakened and morning heart rate.**

- **Night Nogs before bed and bedside if awakened**

- **More frequent and balanced meals**

- **Light exercise**

- **Didn't ignore her cravings for salt.**

  Those concerned with salt relating to high blood pressure can look up the work of Dr. David McCarron and Gary Taubes.

*Sleep is the best meditation.*

— Dalai Lama

# Mary

A week later I was sitting in Mary's large living room. Mary was a fifty-two-year old mother of three who was juggling a career, three teenagers, a busy job, and a sick mother.

"I hear you can work magic," Mary said.

I laughed. "Those allegations have been widely exaggerated, but I understand the magic isn't rubbing off on you too well."

"The Night Nogs you mentioned to Judy have actually helped somewhat."

"Only somewhat?" I questioned.

"Yeah, it's not as frequent, but I still wake up occasionally with high pulse rates, feeling overheated, and usually with my mind spinning," she said.

I had studied her questionnaire earlier that day so I asked, "Would I be correct in assuming you would list mental stress as a key contributor to your present sleep pattern?"

"Without a doubt," she quickly responded.

"Well, the Night Nogs I recommend can help with the 'monkey mind' because lowering adrenaline should have the effect of quieting the mind. Having juice next to your bed so you don't have to get out of bed and make the trek to the kitchen also works very well for clients. The foundation is still built with the Night Nogs."

Mary had told me that one of her main goals was she wanted to sleep better, and therefore wake rested, so she could handle things that "came at her" the next day.

Mary explained, "Back in my twenties I slept like a rock and could go all day with whatever tasks I had to do. But now I struggle to stay awake till 9 p.m., and then wake multiple times during the night. I'm constantly reaching for coffee to keep me going. I feel tired and wired most of the time if that makes sense?"

I nodded.

The lifestyle questionnaire I had emailed Mary two weeks earlier had also revealed her hormonal and mood/thoughts scores were high, which wasn't ideal.

"I have a hard time sleeping with the TV on," she said.

"So why do you have it on?"

Mary rolled her eyes. "Dave, my other half, says he needs to watch the news. Most of the time I wake up with the news still on and buddy boy is asleep."

"The bright flashing light from TV can have an elevating effect on cortisol and an awakening effect not unlike what the sun can do," I said.

"Is that why I sleep better in dark hotel rooms or at the cabin?" she asked.

"Possibly, usually hotel rooms have blackout curtains, but it could also be less electromagnetic stress in the room and especially in the cabin situation. Do you have many electrical devices in your bedroom or a transformer outside your window?" I asked.*

"We have the TV and alarm clock, but no transformer," Mary said.

I added, "If you sleep better somewhere else, then try to find the common denominators."

I asked her to consider if it could be the darkness, the temperature in the room, or the background white noise of the air conditioner.

"We have a loud fan over our bed at the cabin," Mary said.

"That could be it, but I'm guessing it's quiet there anyway," I said.

"It's not. Dave snores when he drinks. If we are at the cabin then he is drinking."

"I can see how the fan may come in handy there," I added.

Mary grinned, "Or the spare bedroom."

"Moving on . . . how's your mattress?" I asked.

"It's a new mattress."

"Could it be more fresh air from being at the cabin? Could it be the lack of noise in a wooded area?" I asked.

"It is quiet there for sure."

"I think it's the light. Our room here isn't dark because of street lights," Mary said as she mentally juggled those questions. "With regard to my hubby's sleeping habits, we can easily put the TV sleep timer on, or the couch will be his new nighttime partner."

Mary was tired of being tired.

"Mary, would it be possible to start dimming lights leading up to bedtime, too?"

"I tend to work at the kitchen table on projects after grade 7 math."

"Grade 7 math?"

"Let's just say I don't think our youngest will be an engineer."

"Gotcha!" I smiled. "In the theme of dimming the lights, I would recommend toning down work related projects if not completely necessary."

"That will be tough. The work is sort of a distraction for me."

"Do you enjoy your work?"

"I have three years, three months, and a few days to retirement," she said.

"I'll take that as a no. The activity should at the very least be something that you enjoy and ideally something that doesn't accelerate the mind or heart rate. Some people use meditation, or yoga, or some other activity centered around a relaxing state which can serve as an unwinding after a fast paced day."

Mary replied, "One of my friends swears by qigong where before she would just swear." We both laughed. "You mean something like that Sean?"

"Basically, anything that doesn't rev the mind up too much," I answered.

The lack of control Mary felt about her mother's situation showed up in something she did have control over which was her work. Many people will use work as a distraction or an avoidance mechanism to an issue they are hesitant to deal with. Nothing is inherently wrong with this, but the avoidance pattern may be energy and vitality consuming, which can deplete a person further.

Society tends to view mental work as beneficial to the brain, but if someone continually exercised their arms with weights, it would eventually be counterproductive. Being able to give yourself mini-mind vacations, like listening to music or a ten to fifteen minute walk in nature, would be a great mental recharger. Rarely does someone return from a nature walk feeling more stressed or fatigued.

*For those concerned about electromagnetic pollution then a EMF meter can be used to detect any above ranges in the house which may disrupt sleeping patterns.

## Breathing

One thing that did stand out in Mary's physical assessment was that her breathing pattern was inverted. Mary was a chest breather instead of breathing diaphragmatically or "belly breathing" as some call it.

"Mary, proper breathing in regard to sleep is something many find beneficial. Breathing shouldn't be complicated, but surprisingly, most breathe incorrectly," I explained. "This can excite the sympathetic nervous system also known as the fight or flight system."

"That doesn't sound like something I want," she said.

"That system is meant for a stressful situation which is polar opposite of sleep. We want you more in the direction of parasympathetic during the night," I said. "Parasympathetic is the part of the autonomic nervous system that helps with digestion, sleep, peristalsis, and more."

"Sean, I never really gave breathing much thought before."

What Mary was doing incorrectly was that on inhaling, she was letting her chest lift and expand, while it should have been moving more in the diaphragm. In other words, if you placed one hand on the upper chest and the other hand over the belly button then which hand moves away from you when you breathe in? It should be the bottom hand feeling like a balloon is being inflated in your stomach upon inhalation.

"Breathing properly through your nose when you first get in bed, and when you wake can have a profound calming effect on the body," I explained.

"That will give me a good excuse to get Dave to turn the TV off. So, what do I do?"

"Practice this first laying down so gravity won't have a profound effect on you. Plus, you are lying down at night so that's where you need it. Once that is perfected, try breathing that way seated and eventually standing. Twelve to sixteen inhalation/exhalation cycles per minute would be good, but ten or less would be optimal. Many clients discover that when they are trying to fall asleep they use a technique called Body Scan used by Jon Kabat-Zinn. The technique involves progressively relaxing your body starting for example, at your toes and working your way up to the top of your head. You spend at least three to four breath cycles on each body part, and with each exhale you focus on relaxing that area progressively. This is a useful technique that can be used if you wake during the night as well," I said.

"Sounds like it would be very relaxing," Mary smiled.

"Indeed, many activities have a focus on breathing like tai chi, qui gong, yoga and martial arts. How we breathe is something we tend to take for granted."

Mary added, "Becoming more of a belly breather shouldn't be hard to fit in the schedule considering I can do that anywhere. Would smoking be the cause of the change in breathing?"

"Smoking could indeed be the etiology of the inverted breathing pattern, but so could a chronic stuffed nose caused by allergies amongst other reasons," I said.

"I had almost stopped smoking, but the present stressors in my life have gotten me increasing my volume," Mary said.

"Breathing pattern problems can result in expelling additional carbon dioxide," I said.

"Carbon dioxide is a bad thing? Right?"

"$CO_2$ is traditionally viewed as a waste product by many in the medical field, but it plays a vital role in pushing oxygen into the cell and has a profound effect on energizing and relaxing the body. An example of this is bag breathing which is an old-school method for people who suffered from panic attacks. The increased level of $CO_2$ in the bag would have a calming effect on the body. Being calm is a great preamble for sleep, don't you think?" I asked.

"Calm is not a word in my vocabulary right now," Mary said, frowning.

"Then that just makes the breathing exercise more of a priority," I encouraged.

"How about drinking water before bed? Is this a good thing to do, or should I avoid it?" Mary wondered. "I have increased my water consumption recently because I believe it helps with my daytime hot flashes," Mary said.

"I'm not saying to ignore your thirst, but if you are getting up a few times a night then you may need to stop or at least reduce water consumption after 6 p.m. If that doesn't change the frequency of waking, then try 3 p.m. If that doesn't change it, then the pelvic floor muscles could be an area of focus."

"You mean like Kegal exercises?" Mary asked.

"They are the ones!"

## Hot Flashes and the Super Carrot

Mary had been having hot flashes over the previous twenty months. She had been drinking six to eight cups of coffee a day, which she agreed to change to either decaf after 3 p.m. or no coffee at all since caffeine after 1 p.m. can disrupt sleep.

"Do you have hot flashes during the day as well?" I questioned.

"Yes, but not as much as the night."

"How is your elimination?" I asked.

"Some days the freight moves and sometimes it's a few days late, if you get my drift," Mary said.

"The amount of elimination can depend on the quantity and quality of food you eat but the frequency can be helped with certain foods," I taught her. "One of the best foods to help this is raw carrots."

"That's something I don't eat much," Mary said.

Raw carrots also will help tremendously to lower estrogen levels. The carrot acts to collect excess estrogen in the bile and bowel so it doesn't get dumped back in the system and cause problems. My clients find that one or two raw carrots daily can take care of all sorts of female hormonal issues within four to six weeks or sooner. The carrots will help immensely, but the body also needs adequate daily protein. A person should aim for at least eighty grams of protein in a day. An example of a daily intake would look like:

Breakfast

2 whole eggs

1 ounce of cheese and 250 grams of milk

Lunch

4 ounces of beef and potato.

Snack 1 ounce of cheese

Supper

16 baby shrimp with a cup of rice and veggies

or steak with root veggies

What I am suggesting can be viewed as big changes for some, but if the desire to change outweighs their present needs, then change will happen.

Five weeks later I received an email from Mary telling me her sleep had greatly improved and she felt rested in the morning. She was having a shredded carrot salad with some olive oil and sea salt. The hot flashes had diminished greatly. She also shifted her water intake to only morning hours and early afternoon.

Lowering her consumption of hot drinks seemed to help her with the daytime hot flashes.

She had also "given herself permission" to do some painting at night. It was a hobby she had enjoyed fifteen years earlier. I had mentioned to her that art work didn't have to be perfect. She wasn't being judged on it so she could even tear it up if she wanted. The purpose was to get the right (parasympathetic) side of the brain involved which serves to relax the body. She was doing this for about ten to fifteen minutes a night. She found it a great way to unwind from the day instead of the distraction of sensationalizing TV or paper work on the kitchen table. She admitted that some nights she would lose track of time while doing her art and almost felt in a meditative state. I never asked about Dave's sleeping accommodations.

TV watching has become the socially accepted meditation and the perceived need to watch the news prior to bed can leave some in a state of despair and restless sleep. Become aware if news and/or TV is having a disruptive impact on your sleep.

## Mary's Keys to Success

- **Night Nogs before and during night if needed**

- **No TV before going to bed and TV sleep timer on**

- **A darker room**

- **Improved breathing mechanics**

- **Limited or no water consumption after 6 p.m.**

- Eating raw carrots daily, leading to improved elimination

- Increased protein

- Mindful activity such as art, tai chi, meditation, slow walking in nature, or funny TV

*Your life is a reflection of how you sleep, and how you sleep is a reflection of your life.*

— Dr. Rafael Pelayo

# Joe

A few weeks passed and I was now in the condo of a client whose paperwork had been reviewed. We were now discussing an obvious blip on his road to health.

"How is your sleep Joe?"

"I call my sleep geographic."

"I have to be honest Joe. I have no idea what you are talking about!"

Joe smiled. "Well - most nights I feel like I'm in the tropics and occasionally I feel like I'm at the North Pole. I'm not sure where I like it better, but at least I get the tropics without the bugs," he said, and laughed.

"Ok now I follow you. Is this a seasonal thing?"

"I'm not sure."

Joe glanced at his phone. "Now that you mention it I believe it is. During the winter my feet and hands are cold a lot. They are cold at night but during the day too."

"How are they in the summer?"

"Not as bad but that doesn't make sense because I have the thermostat set on the same temperature year round in my house and bedroom. But I also tend to wake up sweating and I feel like my heart is coming out through my chest."

"Do you drink alcohol?" I asked.

The question drew his eyes away from his phone.

"Why? Would you like some?" He chuckled. "Yeah, I usually have two or three drinks a night, all depending on what type of day I had," Joe admitted. "Are you going to make me stop drinking because you know how to find your way out." Joe laughed loudly. "I use adult beverages for winding down, especially after I had clients yelling at me all day about their money."

Joe made light of the situation, but I wasn't going to remove something that may have given him a psychological step forward even if it was taking him back physically two steps—yet.

"Stopping is one option but we can try to lessen the alcohol effect on the system first and see if that works. However, we still need you to sleep or you'll just break down at a quicker rate than you are healing. That usually results in what some call vertical disease and then that perpetuates to horizontal disease if you get my drift. Ideally it would be better to avoid the alcohol or reduce the daily volume."

"Break down?" Joe looked puzzled. "Geez, I know I look older than some of my buddies already. I just figured it was my genes, but that makes sense too. That viewpoint shifts the responsibility needle, doesn't it? I'm no stranger to a lot of responsibility," Joe said with a timely look at his phone.

"Joe, you don't have to view it as a burden, but you can look at it as opportunity to have some control over your health. Do you have control over what the stock market does?"

"I wish."

"Doesn't a sense of control feel better than trying to steer a rudderless boat?"

"Yeah, I guess you are right." Joe smiled. "You want a job selling stocks?"

"I don't want to knock you out of a job Joe."

He laughed harder.

"Sean, you know my father died at fifty-nine and I'm almost fifty, so that leaves me with just over 3200 days to live if you take the genetic angle."

Joe could read my face.

"Yeah, I did the math. I do work with numbers all friggin' day remember?"

"Alright Joe, so what do you think you need to do to get on track?"

"Cut out alcohol would be a great first step."

"Is that realistic?" I asked.

"Yeah . . . who's kidding who? Probably not. I know I sound like an alcoholic, but I do go days and weeks without it when I travel and don't miss it. It has become a habit and routine now not unlike when I played squash years ago. It's that addictive personality I'm known for."

Most clients will argue with me that they sleep better with alcohol but I have two questions for them. First, do you wake rested? And second, have you tried a couple of weeks without alcohol to get a benchmark of what your energy really should feel like? The abstinence of alcohol usually brings awareness to what a person's energy levels should resemble.

"Joe, an approach some of my clients take is to have alcohol just on the weekends or only on special occasions which tends to make it just that....special."

Smirking Joe said, "The sun came up today. I think that's special."

"That is true."

"What else can I do?" Joe asked.

I explained that some can have an alcoholic drink with supper with no negative effect. I encouraged Joe to minimize the blood sugar imbalance that can be caused by alcohol by having something fatty like cheese and juice like orange juice before bed to help with blood sugar. I also encouraged him not to drink alcohol on an empty stomach or without food. This may not fix the problem, especially if the quantity is high, but it should lessen those male hot flashes.

"I do get the munchies when I drink alcohol and I usually crave something like potato chips or sweets. How's that for a side plate with wine?" Joe confessed.

"The cravings are extremely common and a prime example of how blood sugar is affected and your body's need to self-regulate," I continued. "The body tends to crave when blood sugar or stored sugar (glycogen) is running low. Something like dark chocolate would be fine but it would be better to reach for some fruit like grapes or cherries and cheese for example."

"I'll have to have keep them stocked in the fridge in that case," Joe said.

"The goal with most of my suggestions is to keep stress minimized. Your cold feet are an example of a stressor than can be fixed by wearing socks to bed."

"My grandmother used to do that. Do I need to wear rollers in my hair too?"

Joe didn't let the conversation stay serious too long.

"Your grandmother was a smart person. Many of my clients also try Epsom salts baths before bed which work very well. Start with three to four cups and don't be afraid of increasing that quantity," I explained.

"I don't like baths, but how about a foot bath?" Joe asked.

"That will work too if you are pressed for time but part of the process of taking a bath is to slow down your pace of life Joe."

"You are a sneaky trainer."

"I wasn't trying to be sneaky, but I was trying to get a feel for your pace of life. If your day consists of constantly living in the fast lane and running at proverbial high rpm's, then it's logical that slowing down at night can be tough but vital if sleep is a priority. So, intentionally taking mini-breaks sort of like mini vacations, even if it's five minutes can serve not only as a recharging of energy but also have a calming effect on the mind and body."

"That makes sense. I guess we get caught up in the more is better mindset," Joe replied.

"I knew you were a smart like your grandmother," I said, smiling at his deep laugh.

Two months later I had a follow up with Joe.

"How's it going Joe? How is your sleep?" I asked with anticipation.

"I would say if I was a new stock then I'd be buying! There has been some trial and error in the process, but overall I'm doing better than I thought." Then Joe added, "I seem to be more focused at work which is unexpected but a welcomed outcome."

"Well most of us get paid to think, so improving the ability to think can reap more than just physical benefits," I said.

"Would better sleep have a positive effect on my mood too?"

"It could. Why?"

"I had a couple of people comment on my good mood over the last few weeks."

"If you sleep better, your energy should be better. And if your energy is better, logic would suggest a better mood," I replied.

"Geez, all along I just thought most people were idiots! Crap, maybe it was just my lack of patience. That's sobering. Which reminds me that I haven't had a drink on a 'school night' since we last met. I had a few cocktails on the weekends, but nothing to the point that the neighbors needed to call the cops."

"I'm sure your neighbors are pleased."

Joe continued, "I initially added some protein and fat alongside the alcohol which for me is usually shellfish and cheese. This did improve the situation some nights, but other nights it didn't. So instead, I changed my after-work ritual. Now when I get home from work around 6 p.m. I have a piece of fruit and some cheese. I then either go for a walk or I go to the gym and do something intense like heavy weights or punching the boxing bag."

"Are you staying with the agreement we discussed in the email?" I asked.

"I am boss," Joe responded. "Like you advised, the days I have energy levels of at least eight out of ten I can push myself towards something more intense. The days that I score lower than that I just take a casual walk," he added.

"Excellent," I said.

Most people seem to think the opposite, believing a stressful day of work should be followed by a more intense workout. This is stress stacked on more stress, and the house of cards grows taller and taller and the likelihood of problems increase.

I made this deal with Joe knowing his personality and that he would like to do everything at full speed. Living in the fast lane of life can be exciting, but the crashes are bigger too.

Joe continued, "The difference this has made is that I don't have the same desire or chance to drink alcohol after work because of my activities. Plus, after exercise, my desire to drink is nonexistent."

"That would be common," I said.

"So, my sleep is better, my energy is improved, and my waistline has even gotten smaller!" Now sticking his thumb inside his belt.

"I would call that a success in my book," I said.

"Now if I could turn myself into a stock I could retire early."

I smiled as Joe laughed again.

A great way to view the human body is on a more global level. An energized cell will relax easier than a tired cell. The common expression, "I couldn't sleep because I was over tired" sums up the problem accurately. You need to give the cell/tissue/organ/muscle/body what it needs for optimal functioning.

The change in Joe's routine coupled with the fact he was exercising enabled him to release stress he may have been carrying. By the end of the walk or workout he didn't have the same desire for alcohol.

The days he walked he felt he slept more soundly, partly due to the exercise but spending time outside in daylight can have a positive effect on the circadian (dark and light) rhythms. The plan for the winter months with his cool feet was to get outside on sunny days. But, he also invested in a 250-watt incandescent bulb which has the appropriate colored (red) wavelength. These bulbs have a calming effect physically and mentally, but also energizes on a cellular level. Along with wearing socks he would use the red-light therapy in the winter evenings or during streaks of grey weather.

The cold hands and feet Joe complained about are typical of blood sugar and adrenaline handling problems, but are also typical of an underactive thyroid. I can't overstate the importance of the thyroid working optimally for proper sleep and ideal health. Thyroid is not excitatory contrary to what some believe. If you view the body as needing energy to function properly, then thyroid would be at the root of the energy source. When I talk about thyroid, I'm referring more towards the active form of thyroid which is T3 (Triiodothyronine) and not T4 (Thyroxine) which is usually all that is tested and prescribed. T4 testing will give a small snapshot of what is happening so other testing may be needed. TSH levels under 2.00 mIU/L should be the goal with lower the better. Testing body temperatures that reach at least 97.8 Fahrenheit or 36.6 Celsius is another simple check of thyroid status. I highly recommend Broda Barnes, Ray Peat, and Mary Shomon for more information on this topic.

Human beings are truly part of nature, so the laws of nature do apply. The human body is intertwined into cyclical patterns such as the seasons and menstrual cycles, and especially day (light) and night (dark). In the summer months, daylight lasts longer and people can manage on less sleep compared to the winter months and still maintain health/energy levels. This seems somewhat instinctive considering how many in the northern hemisphere flock south during the winter months in search of sunshine and heat.

## Joe's Keys to Success

- **Night Nogs**

- **Reduced (or no) alcohol**

- **Wearing socks to bed and/or Epsom salt foot baths**

- **Change of routine (habits) after work**

- **Addition of exercise**

- **Red-light wavelength therapy**

*The body has been as no capacity of lying so listen to what it is saying.*

# Susan

I had just finished with a client at the gym when a woman stood in front of me.

"Are you the trainer?" she asked.

"I am a trainer," I answered.

"I seem to have hit a rut with my training. Can you set me up on a new program?"

"I'd be more than happy to help."

We exchanged information and agreed to be in contact in the next few days.

Susan was a fifty-year-old single mother of three kids looking to "get fit" and maintain her health as she aged. Susan decided she wanted to train at her house and shortly after I arrived she quickly showed me all the equipment she had purchased over the years.

"Do you use these much?" I asked.

"Notice the dust on them?"

Susan's health assessment questionnaire showed hormonal problems, digestive issues, mood and energy swings, and sleep irregularities. Before I could bring up the findings in the questionnaire Susan blurted,

"I have lost 13 pounds in the last 3 months!"

"Intentionally?" I asked.

"What? Yes, of course. I've been running and doing a low carb diet which I have read a few books on. Almost like the Atkins diet I tried years ago. I saw a couple of actresses talking about this diet so I thought I would give it a try. I think I need some weight training added to the program but the diet seems to work great."

"How do you define great?"

"Huh?"

"What is happening that you would define as great?"

"Well, I lost weight and I'm fitting into smaller clothes."

Susan paused.

"I'm not on any medication either," she added sounding unsure if that was an adequate answer.

"Does the questionnaire you filled out reflect how your body has been feeling the last three months?" I asked.

"Yeah, I tried to be accurate," she said.

"Well, it would seem that the questionnaire that you answered may disagree with your definition of great," I said with a smile to let her know she didn't do something wrong.

"Really?" She answered.

"No doubt your weight loss is a great accomplishment, and I'm not trying to minimize it. The questionnaire brings to my attention sleep disturbances, cravings, and hormonal issues."

"I do have those."

"It also shows mood and energy swings. Am I fair in this assessment?"

"Yeah, but most of my friends talk about the same issues."

"It's common," I said.

"And most magazines you read have those articles plastered throughout," Susan said.

"That's true."

"I just assumed when I turned fifty that those things are supposed to happen," Susan said.

"Supposed to happen?" I asked.

"You know change of life - stuff like that. I haven't given it much thought. I just hear about those issues from other people and see them mentioned on TV so frequently that I assumed it was normal," Susan said, shrugging her shoulders.

"It is quite normal to have sleep, energy, and cravings but unfortunately just because it would seem most people experience those things doesn't mean we should experience those things."

"Really?" Susan's eyes were like saucers.

"One of the reasons for the questionnaire is to draw awareness to your health. It may sound cliché, but the absence of sickness does not equal health. When we get our information from heavily sponsored magazines and TV commercials that are selling sickness, we can fall into a misunderstanding of thinking a degree of disease is more the norm," I said.

"Yeah, that seems to be the way," she said. "But I think I look much better than I did three months ago and I seem to have more energy," Susan replied, looking for confirmation.

"I am sure that is indeed the case. The point I'm making is that losing weight is not necessarily synonymous with health and the increased energy could also be artificially driven by adrenaline."

"Driven by adrenaline?"

"This is why I get my clients to monitor their heart rate throughout the day and night to determine if it is indeed adrenaline driven. This takes the guess work out of it," I said.

"Susan, have you slept better or worse in the last three months?" I asked.

"It has been worse. I have a hard time getting to sleep some nights and other nights I awake and can't get back to sleep. Do you think that could be diet related?" Susan asked.

I explained to Susan that when the body is low in fuel (glycogen) our bodies revert to the emergency stress hormones to convert the body into fuel. Your body can turn some protein and fat into fuel, like when on a low carb regime, but it is not the ideal energy source. If the body's need for fuel is not met then the body starts to eat itself by breaking down tissues, organs, and fat which is why the scales move. Unfortunately, destroying tissue and glands along with fat in the process is one step forward and two backwards in the long term with regard to health.

"I definitely don't want my tissues and organs to be eaten," Susan said.

"High on my list to optimizing a person's health will be a focus on getting a person's sleep quality and or quantity towards optimal," I stated. "This results in better energy, better moods, less cravings, less aches and pains, and the ability to do more the next day if desired," I explained.

I continued, saying, "Poor quality sleep will limit your ability to reach any health goal not to mention with fat loss also being hampered. You said you wanted to 'get fit' but that is somewhat a general phrase. I'm not trying to lead you but can you be more specific?" I asked.

"The weight loss is indeed something I like because I have always viewed my appearance as important," Susan said.

"Why?"

"I would have said for health reasons if you asked me that question yesterday."

She paused.

"However, now I'm thinking that those are not analogous. I am guessing it is more to feel good about myself and fit in with my social circle of friends. Geez, I never thought I would say that out loud," she said.

"Susan, they are very real and legitimate reasons."

Susan continued, "My parents always made a fuss over my appearance and the clothes I wore. They would criticize anyone that they deemed fat by calling them lazy or not disciplined. So, I guess I have some of those thoughts buried in me. I also think the media's outlook on health and fitness has been feeding a weed that has been growing a while."

"A weed is a great analogy for those experiences. Your parents did the best they could. All parents do," I said.

"True, they were probably just emulating how they were parented," Susan said.

"This subject may seem off the topic of sleep and health, but all of this is important in addressing the emotional and physical reasons why we are presently living the way we do. Having thoughts of frustration, worry, or inadequacies over appearance can keep people up at night," I said. "Knowing the cause of these thoughts can go a long way in alleviating the problem."

"Susan, with regard to weight (fat) loss I am by no means saying losing weight is a negative. I'm more concerned with the path taken which could be detrimental even with an attractive destination."

"By the way, what time do you exercise?" I asked.

"In the evening from 8:00 to 9:00 p.m."

"That could be a huge factor in your inability to sleep. Intense exercise like running can very stimulating and at that time of day do more harm than good when quality sleep is desired."

"I can move it to an earlier time without a problem."

"Great."

I gave Susan the recipe for the Night Nogs and set her up on a new program.

Three weeks later I was back at Susan's house. Another program was on the agenda, but the topic of sleep had to be discussed.

"Would I be correct in assuming your sleep is better?" I asked.

"Without a doubt," she said. "The orange juice combination was a little hard on my digestion, but the one with just milk and honey worked really well. I slept like a baby the very first night I tried it which is a completely new experience."

"Some people do have digestive problems with orange juice but if they change brands or have it alongside some cheese or other food it seems to help."

"I can try that," Susan replied.

"Adding a pinch of baking soda seems to prevent the digestive issues as well. The orange juice seems to be a more popular pick because it can be quickly put together and some have a mental block with milk and coconut oil," I said.

"My weight has not changed but my energy is much better," Susan said with pride in her voice. "I didn't realize how much my energy had dropped. It was a real mental and physical struggle to exercise while low-carbing but that doesn't seem to be a problem now. Is that the change in food?" Susan asked.

"That could be the result of changing food. Also, the fact that you are sleeping well is important to energy, not to mention mood, mental clarity, and stable blood sugar," I said.

"Susan," I continued. "I was in your position about twenty years ago when I followed muscle mags for advice and ate low carb and high protein. My sleep, joints, and energy were horrible but I dropped weight. My physical appearance didn't match how I felt."

"I guess my health and functioning really does center around sleep!" Susan exclaimed.

"Not sleeping optimally is like building a house in sand. It may hold up for a while but eventually problems will surface. Your sleep, energy, mood, blood sugar, and hormones are very much interdependent of each other. We can sometimes take a reductionist view point and believe they are separate but they hold hands with one another quite intimately," I offered.

"The foundation seems to be laid, so I guess it's time to work on the house and possibly the attic!" Susan chuckled.

## Susan's Keys to Success

- **Night Nogs**

- **Tracking her heart rate**

- **More carbs**

- **Avoiding exercise late in the day**

*In order to get the golden egg you have to take care of the golden goose.*

— Aesop's fable

# What we can learn from these clients

## Client: Judy

### Issues

**Waking during the night (high pulses) and then not being able to fall back to sleep.**

### Takeaway

Judy took a baseline of daily resting heart rate and compared nighttime heart rates. The addition of the Night Nogs shortly before bed helped bring her stress hormones and heart rate down. She used eight to ten ounces of milk with honey and a shake or two of white sea salt (you should not taste the salt). If dairy doesn't agree with you, use fruit juice (tropical ideally). Experiment with adding a teaspoon of coconut oil to the warm milk as well. The oil can have an effect of prolonging the stable blood sugar. The fruit juice should not be from concentrate due to the fact the whole fruit including seeds are usually included in the process and seeds can be problematic on some people's digestion and health.

### Please Note

Sodium intake is a controversial one. Anecdotally everyone's needs seem to be different. Living in hot climates where sweating is common place, or exercising frequently, can cause variations in need. Monitor your fluid intake and excretion. Excretion should be less than half of intake. Please be proactive in your research.

Look at the references I give, but also consult with your doctor and monitor your body's response. Look at all advice with a critical eye. You may want to look into the work of Gary Taubes and David McCarron on the topic.

## Client: Mary

### Issues

- **Waking during the night due to hot flashes**

- **Frequent urination**

- **TV, over-active mind**

- **Inverted breathing**

- **Excess caffeine in the form of coffee or tea in the afternoon**

### Takeaway

Mary implemented a raw carrot salad daily to help rid the body of excess estrogen. Cooked bamboo shoots also serve the same function. She was careful of water and caffeine consumption after 6 p.m. She put on the TV sleep timer, or never turned it on. She had her Night Nogs just before bed which helped quiet the mind. She practiced her slow nose/belly breathing when she got in bed or when she awoke. She also kept a glass of salted orange juice next to the bed in case she woke and felt she couldn't get back to sleep.

Please Note

For those people concerned with excess estrogen (a common cause of hot flashes) should consider the work of Dr. John R. Lee or Dr. Ray Peat. Estrogen blood serum tests only give a picture of what is in the blood and not what is in the tissue.

With respect to the electromagnetic stress, a person can use an EMF field meter to measure any electrical stressors around the bedroom or house which may disrupt sleep.

## Client: Joe

### Issues

- **Waking with heart racing and sweating**

- **Waking in the morning unrested**

- **Cold feet and/or hands frequently in the winter months**

- **Balancing the alcohol's profound effect on blood sugar**

### Takeaway

Changing Joe's routine after work was monumental. The alcohol was a main contributor to the restless nights. Even with the addition of the Night Nogs and food eaten alongside the alcohol, it only seemed to help minimally. Joe realized eliminating or greatly reducing the drinking was the only way to improve his sleep. His change in routine made this change more manageable. The Epsom salt baths had a relaxing effect on the body and along with the socks kept his extremities warm.

# Client: Susan

## Issues

- **Poor sleep**

- **Mood swings**

- **Suboptimal energy**

## Takeaway

Susan would be a person who is praised by others in her peer group due to her weight loss and her change in appearance. Undeniably, the weight loss is an accomplishment. We just need to be conscious of the fact that the mirror and scales don't tell the whole story. If aesthetic goals are solely the prime driver which is extremely common then great. If those aesthetic goals want to be shared with optimal health goals then that is great too. That is a personal decision. Susan avoided exercise late in the day and increased her carbohydrate intake without increasing calories.

A common problem today are dairy intolerances. Try not to always blame the milk considering some have zero problems with dairy. Anybody with this intolerance should start slowly with a couple of ounces and increase over about three to four weeks. Add an ounce each week with food. After the third or fourth week you should be able to handle dairy in larger amounts. Another approach that seems to work is to switch brands or even switch to goat milk. Many allergies result from what the cow has eaten, so simply switching brands can sometimes make a big difference.

A common theme with these four clients, besides the fact they had sleep problems, is that they were willing to make the necessary changes. Sometimes even when the client is paying and asking for help they still do not adhere to the advice. This may be partly due to the mind believing things need to be complex to be effective, or the fact that safety and security are primal needs. Going into the unknown can be scarier for people than where they presently are—even if what they are doing is detrimental.

# Frequently Asked Questions

**1. Can I use something besides orange juice or milk?**

A. Absolutely. This book is meant as a guideline with nothing written in stone. Some clients use other tropical juices like mango, cherry, or pineapple juice or even smoothies. Be aware if the juice causes digestive stress which can happen with apple juice or juice with pulp. I also know others who have just used one or two tablespoons of honey with coconut oil with good results.

**2. The Night Nogs have improved my sleep about 50%. How do I improve more?**

A. The first question to ask yourself is whether it varies and is influenced by your menstrual cycle (days 14–28). If it is, make sure to include raw carrot daily, and to meet protein requirements (eighty grams/day or more). Also, you can turn those Night Nogs into day Nogs. In other words, have them more often and throughout the day (three to four times). The purpose is to keep giving the body what it needs and to maintain consistent energy.

3. **The Night Nogs have given me five hours of continuous sleep where before I would only get three. I still can't fall back to sleep and sometimes it is accompanied with a nightmare. What do I do?**

A. It seems like you are on the right track. Try a nog after supper then another prior to bed. Also have one by the bed and drink it when you wake. Another strategy which may sound counterproductive is alarming the clock twenty to thirty minutes prior to your regular waking time and then having a Nog to "reboot" the sleep pattern. Give it a try for four or five nights and then try no alarm through the night. Some vitamin B supplements cam also give nightmares if taken later in the day.

4. **I'm concerned the salt I added will affect my blood pressure. What do I do?**

A. You always want to check with a medical professional first before making changes. I mentioned previously some do not need the addition of salt to their drinks, while others find it much more beneficial. If there is a history of high blood pressure then it will need to be watched closely. It should be white sea salt and not table salt, and only a pinch is needed for most people. The amount shouldn't be so much that you taste the salt in the drink. Cravings for salt will be a good indicator whether you need more.

5. **Cognitive behavioral therapy (CBT) seems to be a popular recommendation for those with sleep problems. What is your opinion?**

A. CBT has no doubt been effective for many and so has mindfulness-based stress reduction (MBSR). There is no single method that will envelope everybody so the individual with insomnia needs to be proactive with their approach. Like the Night Nogs the treatment is drug-free, so the worst-case scenario is nothing happens.

6. **I have a hard time reaching my daily protein requirements. Can you recommend a protein supplement?**

A. Yes, a great protein supplement would be gelatin. Gelatin consists of various amino acids such as glycine which have been shown to help with sleep. Quality gelatin also doesn't have the additional excipients that most whey proteins carry.

7. **I'm allergic to carrots. Can you recommend something else?**

A. Cooked bamboo shoots will serve the same purpose. Some also use cascara or flowers of sulfer.

## 8. How much juice (Night Nogs) should I have?

A. 4-6 ounces would be a good place to start. If the day has been extra physically and/or emotionally demanding then additional may be required.

## 9. How about melatonin or other supplements?

A. There is no doubt melatonin is effective for some people. The science however, is still weak, so if used, then ideally do so only periodically. Melatonin doesn't result in the same "hangover" as sleeping pills. Supplements such as various forms of magnesium can be helpful. Please experiment with the various brands because I've seen the same brands help one person and bother another.

Hydrolyzed gelatin from a good source can be beneficial. It's tasteless and dissolves in most liquids or goods.

Niacinamide also known as B3 has some anti cortisol and pro metabolic functions, both of which support good sleep. Try to take the B vitamins early in the day. Late in the day can cause nightmares.

Progesterone has also been a supplement that has had great success taken before bed. Progesterone is a tremendous help for many female issues. The ideal brand is Kenogen Progest-E. There are numerous suppliers depending on your location. Don't confuse it with progestin.

**10. You mentioned thyroid as an underlying issue. If my blood tests are "normal," then what do I do?**

A. Thyroid is a major player. Blood serum levels will give some idea to what's happening. It still doesn't reveal what is in the tissue, however. TSH levels under 2.0 are optimal. The lower the better. You may be told it's good at 3.2, but your body will say otherwise. Body temperatures of at least 36.6 Celsius or 97.8 Fahrenheit is one simple home test you can use for checking. Take your temperature for three to four days and the average should be over 97.8. Chronically cold extremities is a common symptom of an under active thyroid.

**11. I like to read in bed on my tablet which puts me in a good head space to fall asleep. Is there anything to help with the light from the phone or tablet?**

A. Yes, there is. You can download the app F.lux which reduces the blue light emitted from these devices. Blue light wavelength has been linked to adverse health problems and poor sleep.

# Night Nogs

## Options

- Six to eight ounces of white milk, and a couple shakes of White Sea salt. Optional: add a teaspoon of unflavored coconut oil with enough hot water to melt the oil

- Orange juice, not from concentrate, with no pulp, and a couple shakes of white sea salt (there is no need to taste the salt for effectiveness)

- Half milk and half orange juice with a couple shakes of white sea salt

- If orange juice irritates the stomach then either use ¼ teaspoon of baking soda to lower the acidity or try another brand that agrees with you. You could also try another tropical juice like pineapple or mango

- Six to eight ounces of milk with a teaspoon or two of honey

- Others have used ice cream as well, but do check the label for additives such as carrageenan, and other gums like guar and bean

*Good sleep requires fairly vigorous metabolism and a normal body temperature. In old age, the metabolic rate is decreased, and sleep becomes defective.*

— Ray Peat, PhD

# Checklist

- Night Nogs are the most important aspect

- Drink Nogs before bed and have bedside if awakened

- Reduce or eliminate caffeine after 1 p.m.

- Reduce or eliminate alcohol

- Minimize physical and mental stimulating activities after supper

- Reduce or eliminate water consumption after supper or earlier if needed

- Create a smooth transition to bed such as: dimming lights, taking bath, watching funny T.V. reading light material and avoid stressful work or stimulating, disturbing T.V.

- Keep extremities warm with socks, hot water bottles, and long pajamas. Epsom salt baths before bed are great

- Daily sunshine or red-light wavelength therapy during the winter months

- Raw carrots daily especially if cycle related or menopausal related. Normal bowel functioning is extremely important

- Compare awakened heart rate to resting heart rate to determine if adrenaline driven. If adrenaline, then more Nogs are needed

- Diaphragmatic breathing, especially when trying to get to sleep

- Grazing throughout the day to keep blood sugar levels stable

- Get enough daily protein (80 grams or more)

- Try to maintain the same bedtime

- Use F. lux software to protect from blue light

- Keep bedroom environment suitable for sleep such as darkness, noise, temperature, etc.

- Exercise every day. It doesn't have to be intense—just move. Walking is nature would be great

- Optimal thyroid functioning

- Do something you enjoy every day

Please try these suggestions and let me know your progress. These recommendations are typically fast acting from the first night of implementation, to about six weeks. Thank you for taking your time to read the book. I know you are on your way to restoring your sleep!

*The starting point of all achievement is desire.*

- Napolean Hill

Good luck and stay well,

Sean Mullowney

LifeRightSideUp.com

Sean@LifeRightSideUp.com

# References

1.  Sugar lowering stress

    http://www.functionalps.com/blog/2011/02/04/sugar-sucrose-restrains-the-stress-hormone-system/

2.  Salt

    http://www.functionalps.com/blog/2012/08/21/sodium-deficiency-and-stress/

3.  Winter deaths

    http://www5.statcan.gc.ca/cansim/a05?lang=eng&id=1020502

4.  Low salt and poor sleep

    http://www.ncbi.nlm.nih.gov/pubmed

5.  Potassium

    Chatterjee JR. Serum and Dietary Potassium and Risk of Incident Type 2 Diabetes Mellitus. Arch Int Med 2010; 170(19):1745-1751

6.  Fructose -Nilsson, L. H., & Hultman, E. (1974). Liver and muscle glycogen in man after glucose and fructose infusion. Scandinavian journal of clinical and laboratory investigation, 33(1), 5–10. Retrieved from

    http://www.ncbi.nlm.nih.gov/pubmed/

7. EMF

   http://www.ncbi.nlm.nih.gov/pubmed/10188140

8. Breathing and autonomic system

   http://www.ncbi.nlm.nih.gov/pubmed/15347862

9. Co2 sedative effect

   http://www.ncbi.nlm.nih.gov/pubmed/7675582

10. magnesium and sleep

    http://www.ncbi.nlm.nih.gov/pubmed/11777170

    http://www.ncbi.nlm.nih.gov/pubmed/8232845

12. Sunlight

    Peat, R. (1996). Using Sunlight to Sustain Life. Townsend Letter for Doctors & Patients, (155), 83

13. Sleep and cravings

    http://www.nature.com/ncomms/2013/130806/ncomms3259/full/ncomms3259.html

14. Glycine and sleep

    Sleep and Biological rhythms, 2007 5(2), 126-131. Glycine ingestion improves subjective sleep quality in human volunteers, correlating with polysomnographic changes. Yamadera W, Inagawa K, Chiba S, Bannai M, Takahashi M, Nakayama K

Sleep and Biological Rhythms 2006 4(1), 75-77. Subjective effects of glycine ingestion before bedtime on sleep quality. Inagawa K, Hiraoka T, Kohda T, Yamadera W, Takahashi M.

**Further resources**

http://raypeat.com/

http://www.brodabarnes.org/

http://www.johnleemd.com/

http://garytaubes.com/wp-content/uploads/2011/08/science-political-science-of-salt.pdf

http://www.stevenhalpern.com/relaxintosleep

https://www.mindfulnesscds.com/

https://redlightman.com/blog/

# About Author

Sean Mullowney started his personal training business in 1996. He has accumulated more than 30,000 client hours. He has worked with clients ranging in various abilities. From a professional hockey team and Olympic medalist to weekend warriors and those in need of rehab.

Sean studied Exercise Science at Concordia University and is 1 of 5 Chek Level 3 practitioners in Canada. He is the only Holistic Lifestyle Coach Level 3 in Atlantic Canada.

Sean is also a naturopath.